# AIR FRYER

## Cookbook for Beginners

*Snack*

*Dessert Recipes*

**SOPHIA SMITH**

# Table of Contents

—
4

# Disclaimer Notice:

Please note the information contained within this document is for educational and entertainment purposes only. All effort has been executed to present accurate, up to date, and reliable, complete information. No warranties of any kind are declared or implied. Readers acknowledge that the author is not engaging in the rendering of legal, financial, medical or professional advice. The content within this book has been derived from various sources. Please consult a licensed professional before attempting any techniques outlined in this book.By reading this document, the reader agrees that under no

 circumstances is the author responsible for any losses, direct or indirect, which are incurred as a result of the use of information contained within this document, including, but not limited to, errors, omissions, or inaccuracies.

# Introduction:

The air fryer is an essential device that caused many people to think about healthy food or healthy cooking. The Air fryer is the right way to use the regular pan or other fryers because it doesn't have oil that makes your cooking extra fat. Besides that, the air fryer is so easy to be cleaned. There is no oily residue that will stick on the deep fryer after use. No smoke or scent will stay in the kitchen after use. The air fryer has its merit that people can try it. An air fryer is a gadget that helps you fry your meals by circulating air around the meal. The air is heated to the required temperature of the food that you want to deep fry. This way, the food will not have to be soaked in oil.

You should know that you will still taste delicious of your food like it makes crunchy after cooking. You could choose to put different vegetables or meat on it and turn it into a complete meal.

The air fryer has many benefits for you so that you can enjoy the air fryer more. First, it will help you to save time by cooking food for your family and friends can enjoy. It is a perfect fit for a small kitchen, and it can be used on many occasions, such as the birthday cake. It will be a special day for you, and you will not just cook the same cake but make it a little bit more special for your special day. Second, it is very easy to be stored. It is very safe for your children because this is an extra safety, so it will not be dangerous. The fryer is so light that you can bring it with you as a traveling bag. It is so easy to clean. You do not have to think about the safety of your children when you cook with the air fryer. You can also find a lot of recipes with the air fryer. You can cook using this tool many different things, such as chicken, fish, and so on. It has all the time you need, and you do not need to repeat cooking if you have to cook multiple dishes. It is very easy to be all over. Third, it will make your food to be cooked fast, and it can be enjoyed easily. The food will be cooked quickly, and there is no need to wait so long for your food to be cooked. It just likes the regular fryer that you use in your kitchen. The food will be cooked as you wait.Finally, it can be used on many occasions. You can use it more than you think. This is the right thinking because this device has the merit that you can use it in many places. On special occasions, you can use this fryer for a cooking cake for the word of your own. It will be a romantic feeling for sure, and you can use this for cooking even when you are in a small place. The Air fryer is the right choice for you. The Air fryer is made by a person who has excellent experience the fried food, but he also has a great idea to make healthy fried food for people who want to keep their healthy lifestyle and eat as good as possible. This idea makes many people start to love the Air fryer because it is perfect for them. Some people begin to try and begin to love the fried food for their body and health. But how can the air fryer make healthy food? The air fryer is excellent cooking equipment for a healthy diet. Many people think that fried food is tasty, but it is not healthy. Using the air frying process, it is possible to prepare different types of raw food in a healthy way. Many scientific researchers say that a healthy diet is very important for our life now. It helps us to have a healthy body and maintain nutrition for all body parts. An air fryer utilizes the worthlessness of energy to make tasty food.

Use the Air fryer but to make healthier food, you need to know the basic way of using it.

You need to understand the setting, how you can change the heating setting, and set the temperature for your food frying.

This air fryer uses the fan and heating element, making the baked food have no greasy and fried smell like deep frying the food. To use this air fryer, you need to heat the food for a little while, then put the food over the air fryer, transfer the temperature between the foods and keep the temperature stable even if you shut off the heat.

You need to spray the oil over the air fryer and the food surface you cook. It can be helpful to use the proper oil spray can for convenience if you want. The oil needs to cover the entire body because the Air fryer needs to reheat the food through the bottom and top. If you do not cover, the fish or chicken will burn on the sides due to the opening.

You only need to half the food to 300 degrees F. If you are trying to cook a large piece, reduce the temperature for your large amount.

You need to keep the cooked food aside if the food is not cooked yet when you will be transferring the temperature. Always keep the oven door closed to avoid any odor, and always use the clean container to keep the food.

# Snack

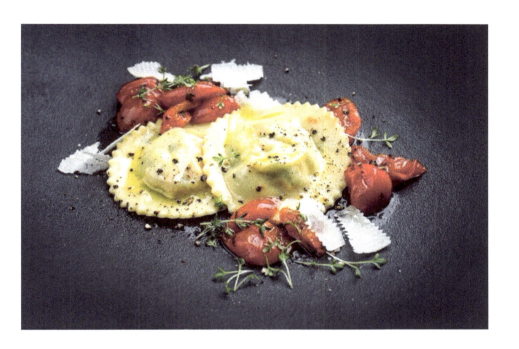

# 1. Sweet Potato Tater Tots

Preparation Time: 10 minutes

Cooking Time: 23 minutes

Serving 4

## Ingredients:

- Two sweet potatoes, peeled
- 1/2 tsp. Cajun seasoning
- Olive oil cooking spray
- Sea salt to taste

## Directions:

1. Boil sweet potatoes in water for 15 minutes over medium-high heat. Drain the sweet potatoes, then allow them to cool.

2. Peel the boiled sweet potatoes and return them to the bowl. Mash the potatoes and stir in salt and Cajun seasoning. Mix well and make small tater tots out of it. Place the tater tots in the Air Fryer basket and spray them with cooking oil.

3. Set the Air Fryer basket inside the Air Fryer toaster oven and close the lid. Select the Air Fry mode at 400°F temperature for 8 minutes. Flip the tater tots and continue cooking for another 8 minutes. Serve fresh.

**Nutrition:**

Calories: 184 Cal

Protein: 9 g

Carbs: 43 g

Fat: 17 g

## 2. Fried Ravioli

Preparation Time: 10 minutes

Cooking Time 15 minutes

Serves: 4

**Ingredients:**

- One package ravioli, frozen

- 1 cup breadcrumbs

- 1/2 cup parmesan cheese

- One tbs. Italian seasoning

- One tbs. garlic powder

- Two eggs, beaten

- Cooking spray

**Directions:**

1. Mix breadcrumbs with garlic powder, cheese, and Italian seasoning in a bowl. Whisk eggs in another bowl.

2. Dip each ravioli in eggs first, then coat them with a crumbs mixture. Place the ravioli in the Air Fryer

basket. Set the Air Fryer basket inside the Air Fryer toaster oven and close the lid. Select the Air Fry mode at 360°F temperature for 15 minutes.

3. Flip the ravioli after 8 minutes and resume cooking. Serve warm.

**Nutrition:**

Calories: 124 Cal

Protein: 4.5 g

Carbs: 27.5 g

Fat: 3.5 g

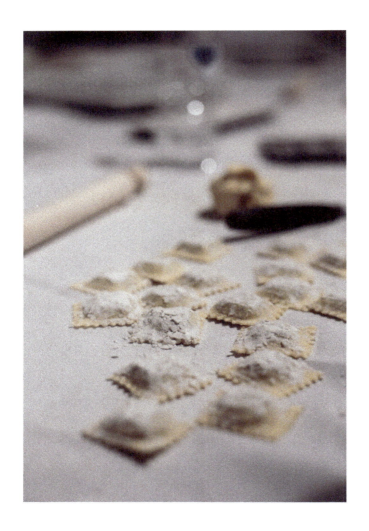

# 3. Eggplant Fries

Preparation Time: 10 minutes

Cooking Time 20 minutes

Serves: 4

## Ingredients:

- 1/2 cup panko breadcrumbs

- 1/2 tsp. salt

- One eggplant, peeled and sliced

- 1 cup egg, whisked

## Directions:

1. Toss the breadcrumbs with salt in a tray. Dip the eggplant in the whisked egg and coat with the crumb's mixture. Place the eggplant slices in the Air Fryer basket.

2. Set the Air Fryer basket inside the Air Fryer toaster oven and close the lid. Select the Air Fry mode at 400°F temperature for 20 minutes. Flip

the slices after 10 minutes, then resume cooking.

Serve warm.

## Nutrition:

Calories: 110 Cal

Protein: 5 g

Carbs: 12.8 g

Fat: 11.9 g

# 4. Stuffed Eggplants

Preparation Time: 10 minutes

Cooking Time 38 minutes

Serves: 4

## Ingredients:

- Two eggplants, cut in half lengthwise

- 1/2 cup shredded cheddar cheese

- 1/2 can (7.5 oz.) chili without beans

- 2 tsp. kosher salt

For Serving

- 2 tbsp. cooked bacon bits

- 2 tbsp. sour cream

- Fresh scallions, thinly sliced

## Directions:

1. Place the eggplant halves in the Air Fryer basket. Set the basket inside the Air Fryer toaster oven and close the lid. Select the Air Fry mode at 390°F temperature for 35 minutes.

2. Top each eggplant half with chili, cheese, and salt. Place the halves in a baking pan and return to the oven.

3. Select the Broil mode at 375°F temperature for 3 minutes. Garnish with bacon bits, sour cream, and scallions. Serve.

**Nutrition:**

Calories: 113 Cal

Protein: 9.2 g

Carbs: 13 g

Fat: 21 g

# 5. Bacon Poppers

Preparation Time: 10 minutes

Cooking Time 15 minutes

Serves: 4

## Ingredients:

- Four strips bacon, crispy cooked

Dough:

- 2/3 cup water

- 3 tbsp. butter

- 1tbsp. bacon fat

- 1tsp. kosher salt

- 2/3 cup all-purpose flour

- Two eggs

- 2 oz. Cheddar cheese, shredded

- ½ cup jalapeno peppers

- A pinch pepper

- A pinch black pepper

## Directions:

1. Whisk butter with water and salt in a skillet over medium heat. Stir in flour, then stir cook for about 3 minutes. Transfer this flour to a bowl, then whisk in eggs and the rest of the ingredients. Fold in bacon and mix well.

2. Wrap this with dough in a plastic sheet and refrigerate for 30 minutes. Make small balls out of this dough. Place these bacon balls in the Air Fryer basket. Set the basket inside the Air Fryer toaster oven and close the lid. Select the Air Fry mode at 390°F temperature for 15 minutes. Flip the balls after 7 minutes, then resume cooking. Serve warm.

## Nutrition:

Calories: 240 Cal

Protein: 14.9 g

Carbs: 7.1 g

Fat: 22.5 g

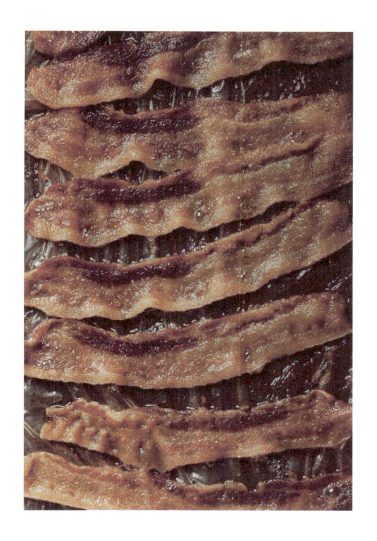

# 6. Stuffed Jalapeno

Preparation Time: 10 minutes

Cooking Time 10 minutes

Serves: 4

## Ingredients:

- 1 lb. ground pork sausage

- 1 (8 oz.) package cream cheese, softened

- 1 cup shredded Parmesan cheese

- 1 lb. sizeable fresh jalapeno peppers halved lengthwise and seeded

- 1 (8 oz.) bottle Ranch dressing

## Directions:

1. Mix pork sausage ground with ranch dressing and cream cheese in a bowl. But the jalapeno in half and remove their seeds. Divide the cream cheese mixture into the jalapeno halves. Place the jalapeno pepper in a baking tray.

2. Set the Baking tray inside the Air Fryer toaster oven and close the lid. Select the Bake mode at 350°F temperature for 10 minutes. Serve warm.

**Nutrition:**

Calories: 168 Cal

Protein: 9.4 g

Carbs: 12.1 g

Fat: 21.2 g

# 7. Creamy Mushrooms

Preparation Time: 10 minutes

Cooking Time 15 minutes

Serves: 24

## Ingredients:

- 20 mushrooms
- One orange bell pepper, diced
- One onion, diced
- Three slices bacon, diced
- 1 cup shredded Cheddar cheese
- 1 cup sour cream

## Directions:

1. First, sauté the mushroom stems with onion, bacon, and bell pepper in a pan.
2. After 5 minutes of cooking, add 1 cup cheese and sour cream—Cook for 2 minutes.
3. Place the mushroom caps on the Air Fryer basket crisper plate.

4. Stuff each mushroom with the cheese-vegetable mixture and top them with cheddar cheese.

5. Insert the basket back inside and select Air Fry mode for 8 minutes at 350°F.

6. Serve warm.

**Nutrition:**

Calories: 101 Cal

Protein: 8.8 g

Carbs: 25 g

Fat: 12.2 g

# 8. Italian Corn Fritters

Preparation Time: 10 minutes

Cooking Time 3 minutes

Serves: 4

**Ingredients:**

- 2 cups frozen corn kernels
- 1/3 cup finely ground cornmeal
- 1/3 cup flour
- ½ tsp. salt
- ¼ tsp. pepper
- ½ tsp. baking powder
- Onion powder, to taste
- Garlic powder, to taste
- ¼ tsp. paprika
- 2 tbsp. green chilies with juices
- 3 tbsp. almond milk
- ¼ cup chopped Italian parsley

## Directions:

1. Beat cornmeal with flour, baking powder, parsley, seasonings in a bowl. Blend 3 tbsp. Almond milk with 1 cup corn, black pepper, and salt in a food processor until smooth. Stir in the flour mixture, then mix until smooth.

2. Spread this corn mixture in a baking tray lined with wax paper. Set the baking tray inside the Air Fryer toaster oven and close the lid. Select the bake mode at 350°F temperature for 2 minutes. Slice and serve.

## Nutrition:

Calories: 146 Cal

Protein: 6.3 g

Carbs: 18.8 g

Fat: 4.5 g

# 9. Artichoke Fries

Preparation Time: 8 minutes

Cooking Time 13 minutes

Serves: 6

**Ingredients:**

- 1 oz. can artichoke hearts

- 1 cup flour

- 1 cup almond milk

- ½ tsp. garlic powder

- ¾ tsp. salt

- ¼ tsp. black pepper, or to taste

For Dry Mix:

- ½ cup panko breadcrumbs

- ½ tsp. paprika

- ¼ tsp. salt

## Directions:

1. Whisk the wet ingredients in a bowl until smooth and mix the dry ingredients in a separate bowl. First, dip the artichokes quarters in the wet mixture, then coat with the dry panko mixture.

2. Place the artichokes hearts in the Air Fryer basket. Set the Air Fryer basket inside the Air Fryer toaster oven and close the lid. Select the Air Fry mode at 340°F temperature for 13 minutes. Serve warm.

## Nutrition:

Calories: 199 Cal

Protein: 9.4 g

Carbs: 15.9 g

Fat: 4 g

# 10.    Crumbly Beef Meatballs

Preparation Time: 8 minutes

Cooking Time 20 minutes

Serves: 6

**Ingredients:**

- 2lbs. of ground beef

- 2large eggs

- 1-1/4 cup panko breadcrumbs

- 1/4 cup chopped fresh parsley

- 1 tsp. dried oregano

- 1/4 cup grated Parmigianino Reggiano

- One small clove of garlic chopped

- salt and pepper to taste

- 1 tsp. vegetable oil

## Directions:

1. Thoroughly mix beef with eggs, crumbs, parsley, and the rest of the ingredients.

2. Create small meatballs out of this mixture and place them in the Air Fryer basket. Set the basket inside the Air Fryer toaster oven and close the lid.

3. Select the Air Fry mode at 350°F temperature for 13 minutes. Toss the meatballs after 5 minutes and resume cooking. Serve fresh.

## Nutrition:

Calories: 221 Cal

Protein: 25.1 g

Carbs: 11.2 g

Fat: 16.5 g

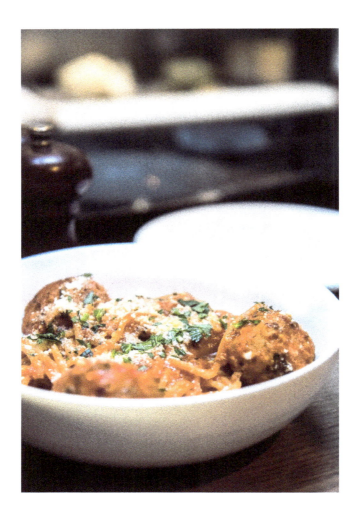

# 11.   Pork Stuffed Dumplings

Preparation Time: 15 minutes

Cooking Time 12 minutes

Serves: 3

**Ingredients:**

- 1 tsp. canola oil

- 4 cups chopped book Choy

- 1 tbsp. chopped fresh ginger

- 1 tbsp. chopped garlic

- 4 oz. ground pork

- 1/4 tsp. crushed red pepper

- 18 dumpling wrappers

- Cooking spray

- 2 tbsp. rice vinegar

- 2 tsp. Lower-sodium soy sauce

- tsp. toasted sesame oil

- 1/2 tsp. packed light Sugar

- 1 tbsp. finely chopped scallions

**Directions**:

1. In a greased skillet, sauté bok choy for 8 minutes, then add ginger and garlic. Cook for 1 minute. Transfer the bok choy to a plate.

2. Add pork and red pepper, then mix well. Place the dumpling wraps on the working surface and divide the pork fillings on the dumpling wraps. Wet the edges of the wraps and pinch them together to seal the filling.

3. Place the dumpling in the Air Fryer basket. Set the Air Fryer basket inside the Air Fryer toaster oven and close the lid. Select the Air Fry mode at 375°F temperature for 12 minutes. Flip the dumplings after 6 minutes, then resume cooking. Serve fresh.

## Nutrition:

Calories: 172 Cal

Protein: 2.1 g

Carbs: 18.6 g

Fat: 10.7 g

# 12.    Panko Tofu with Mayo Sauce

Preparation Time: 10 minutes

Cooking Time 20 minutes

Serves: 4

**Ingredients:**

- Eight tofu cutlets

For the Marinade

- tbsp. toasted sesame oil

- 1/4 cup soy sauce

- 1 tsp. rice vinegar

- 1/2 tsp. garlic powder

- 1 tsp. ground ginger

Make the Tofu:

- 1/2 cup vegan mayo

- cup panko breadcrumbs

- 1 tsp. of sea salt

## Direction:

1. Whisk the marinade ingredients: in a prepared bowl and add tofu cutlets. Mix well to coat the cutlets. Cover and marinate for 1 hour. Meanwhile, whisk crumbs with salt and mayo in a bowl. Coat the cutlets with crumbs mixture.

2. Place the tofu cutlets in the Air Fryer basket. Set the basket inside the Air Fryer toaster oven and close the lid. Select the Air Fry mode at 370°F temperature for 20 minutes. Flip the cutlets after 10 minutes, then resume cooking. Serve warm.

## Nutrition:

Calories: 151 Cal

Protein: 1.9 g

Carbs: 6.9 g

 Fat: 8.6 g

# 13.   Garlicky Bok Choy

Preparation Time: 10 minutes

Cooking Time 10 minutes

Serves: 2

## Ingredients:

- Four bunches baby book Choy

- Spray oil

- tsp. garlic powder

## Directions:

1. Toss bok choy with garlic powder and spread them in the Air Fryer basket. Spray them with cooking oil. Place the basket inside the Air Fryer toaster oven and close the lid. Select the Air Fry mode at 350°F temperature for 6 minutes. Serve fresh.

## Nutrition:

Calories: 81 kcal

Protein: 0.4 g

Carbs: 4.7 g

Fat: 8.3 g

# 14. Seasoned Cauliflower Chunks

Preparation Time: 10 minutes

Cooking Time 15 minutes

Serves: 4

**Ingredients:**

- One cauliflower head, diced into chunks

- ½ cup unsweetened milk

- 6 tbsp. mayo

- ¼ cup all-purpose flour

- ¾ cup almond meal

- ¼ cup almond meal

- tsp. onion powder

- 1 tsp. garlic powder

- 1 tsp. of sea salt

- ½ tsp. paprika

- Pinch of black pepper

- Cooking oil spray

## Directions:

1. Toss cauliflower with the rest of the ingredients in a bowl, then transfers to the Air Fryer basket. Spray them with cooking oil. Set the basket inside the Air Fryer toaster oven and close the lid. Select the Air Fry mode at 400°F temperature for 15 minutes. Toss well and serve warm.

## Nutrition:

Calories: 137 Cal

Protein: 6.1 g

Carbs: 26 g

Fat: 8 g

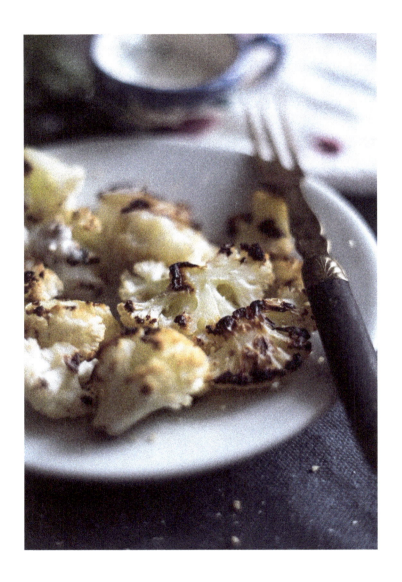

# 15.    Tofu Popcorns

Preparation Time: 15 minutes

Cooking Time 15 minutes

Serves: 4

**Ingredients:**

- 2 cups tofu, diced
- Three ¾ cups vegetable broth, divided
- Two garlic cloves, mashed
- tsp. salt
- 1-inch cube ginger, grated
- ½ cup all-purpose flour
- ½ cup of corn starch
- cup panko breadcrumbs
- 1 tbsp. garlic powder
- 1 tbsp. lemon pepper
- ½ tsp. salt

## Directions:

1. Toss tofu with ginger, salt, and garlic in a large bowl. Pour in 3 cups of broth and soak for 20 minutes. Whisk wheat flour with cornstarch and ¾ cup broth in a bowl until smooth. Remove the tofu cubes from the milk and dip the cubes in the flour batter.

2. Place the tofu chunks in the Air Fryer basket. Set the basket inside the Air Fryer toaster oven and close the lid. Select the Air Fry mode at 390°F temperature for 15 minutes. Serve fresh.

## Nutrition:

Calories: 110 Cal

Protein: 2.7 g

Carbs: 12.8g

Fat: 1.9 g

# 16.    Cauliflower Tater Tots

Preparation Time: 15 minutes

Cooking Time 10 minutes

Serves: 6

**Ingredients:**

- 1-pound fresh cauliflower, cut into chunks

- tbsp. Cheddar cheese

- cup Panko breadcrumbs

- tsp. desiccated coconut

- tsp. Oats

- One egg, beaten

- tbsp. onion, chopped

- tsp. garlic puree

- 1 tsp. parsley

- 1 tsp. chives

- 1 tsp. oregano

- Salt and pepper to taste

## Directions:

1. Boil the fresh cauliflower florets in salted water for 10 minutes until soft, then drain. Mash the cauliflower in a bowl and then stir in salt, black pepper, garlic, parsley, chives, and oregano. Mix well, and then make small tater tots out of this mixture. Mix breadcrumbs with oats and coconut shreds in a tray.

2. Dip the tater tots in the egg, then coat with the crumb's mixture. Place the tater tots in the Air Fryer basket. Place the basket inside the Air Fryer toaster oven and close the lid. Select the Air Fry mode at 360°F temperature for 10 minutes. Serve warm and fresh.

## Nutrition:

Calories: 121 Cal

Protein: 12.8 g

Carbs: 35.2 g

Fat: 6.6 g

# 17.   Cauliflower Patties

Preparation Time: 10 minutes

Cooking Time 20 minutes

Serves: 4

**Ingredients:**

- Three large eggs
- 3 cups cauliflower florets
- ½ cup all-purpose flour
- 3 tbsp. wheat flour
- tsp. coconut oil (melted)
- ½ tsp. garlic powder
- ½ tsp. turmeric
- ½ tsp. parsley
- Salt & pepper to taste
- Cooking oil spray

**Directions:**

1. Grate the cauliflower in a food processor; add parsley, turmeric, garlic powder, and wheat flour. Whisk in eggs, and coconut oil, then mix well. Make four patties out of this cauliflower mixture and place them in the Air Fryer basket.

2. Set the Air Fryer basket inside the Air Fryer toaster oven and close the lid. Select the Air Fry mode at 375°F temperature for 20 minutes. Serve warm.

**Nutrition:**

Calories: 110 Cal

Protein: 1.8g

Carbs: 14.3 g

Fat: 5.6 g

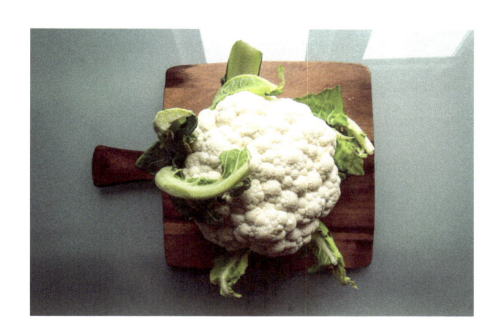

# 18.    Tilapia Fish Sticks

Preparation Time: 10 minutes

Cooking Time 15 minutes

Serves: 4

**Ingredients:**

- Four frozen tilapia fillets, cut into sticks
- cup all-purpose flour
- Two large eggs, beaten
- 1/2 cups seasoned panko breadcrumbs
- 1 tbsp. kosher salt

For serving:

- One lemon, cut in wedges
- Tartar sauce
- Ketchup

## Directions:

1. Mix flour with salt and dredge the tilapia sticks through the flour, then dip them in the egg and finally coat with the crumb's mixture. Place the coated bars in the Air Fryer basket. Set the basket inside the Air Fryer toaster oven and close the lid.

2. Select the Air Fry mode at 390°F temperature for 12 minutes. Serve with lemon wedges, tartar sauce, and ketchup.

## Nutrition:

Calories: 283 Cal

Protein: 20.3 g

 Carbs: 12 g

Fat: 10.2 g

# 19.    Bacon-Wrapped Scallops

Preparation Time: 10 minutes

Cooking Time 12 minutes

Serves: 9

## Ingredients:

- ½ cup mayonnaise

- 2 tbsp. Sriracha sauce

- 1-pound bay scallops

- pinch coarse salt

- One pinch freshly cracked black pepper

- 12 slices bacon, cut into three pieces

- Olive oil cooking spray

## Directions:

1. Whisk Sriracha sauce with mayonnaise in a bowl and keep it aside. Place the scallops on the working surface and pat them dry. Sprinkle some salt and black pepper on top, then wrap the 1/3 of a bacon slice around the scallops and secure it

by inserting a toothpick. Place the scallops on the Air Fryer basket.

2.  Put the basket inside the Air Fryer toaster oven and close the lid. Select the Air Fry mode at 390°F temperature for 7 minutes. Serve warm with mayo sauce.

**Nutrition:**

Calories: 222 Cal

Protein: 17.3 g

Carbs: 3.3 g

Fat: 15.3 g

# Dessert Recipes

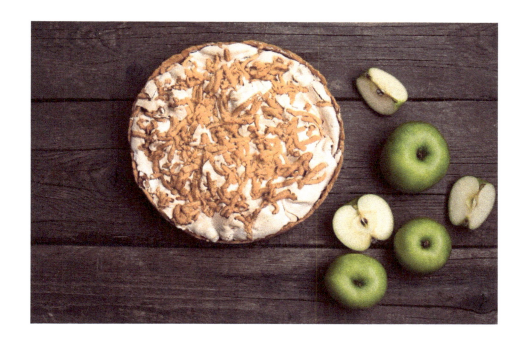

# 20.   Dessert Vanilla French toast

Preparation Time: 5 minutes

Cooking Time: 4 minutes

Servings: 4

## Ingredients:

- One egg whisked

- 1/4 cup coconut milk

- 2 tbsp. butter, melted

- tsp. vanilla paste

- 1/2 tsp. ground cinnamon

- A pinch of grated nutmeg

- slices bread

## Directions:

1. In a mixing bowl, thoroughly combine the eggs, milk, butter, vanilla, cinnamon, and nutmeg.

2. Then dip each piece of bread into the egg mixture; place the bread slices in a lightly greased baking pan.

3. Air Fryer the bread slices at 330 degrees F for about 4 minutes; flip and cook for 3 to 4 minutes. Enjoy!

**Nutrition:**

Calories 164

Fat 10.4g

Carbs 11.7g

Protein 4.6g

Fiber 0.8g

# 21.    Street-Style Spanish Churros

Preparation Time: 10 minutes

Cooking Time: 10 minutes

Servings: 4

**Ingredients:**

- 3/4 cup all-purpose flour

- 1/2 tsp. baking powder

- 3/4 cup water

- 4 tbsp. butter

- 1 tbsp. granulated sugar

- 1/2 tsp. vanilla extract

- 1/2 tsp. sea salt

- One large egg

**Directions:**

1. In a prepared mixing bowl, thoroughly combine all ingredients. In a piping bag equipped with a wide open star tip, put the batter.

2. Pipe the churros into 6-inch long ropes and lower them onto the greased Air Fryer pan.

3. Cook your churros in the preheated Air Fryer at 360 degrees F for 10 minutes, flipping them halfway through the cooking time.

4. Repeat the process use the remaining batter and then serve warm. Enjoy!

## Nutrition:

214 Calories

12.4g Fat

20.1g Carbs

4.4g Protein

0.6g Fiber

# 22.    Vanilla-Cinnamon Pears in Wine

Preparation Time: 3 minutes

Cooking Time: 17 minutes

Servings: 3

## Ingredients:

- Three pears, peeled and cored
- One vanilla pod
- One cinnamon stick
- 2-3 cloves
- cup caster sugar
- 1 cup red wine

## Directions:

1. Place the pears, vanilla, cinnamon, cloves, sugar, and wine in an Air Fryer safe dish.
2. Cook the pears at 340 degrees F for 17 minutes.
3. Serve at room temperature. Bon appétit!

## **Nutrition:**

185 Calories

0.2g Fat

47.1g Carbs

1g Protein

4.4g Fiber

# 23.  Coconut Chocolate Cake

Preparation Time: 5 minutes

Cooking Time: 20 minutes

Servings: 6

**Ingredients:**

- 1/2 cup coconut oil, room temperature
- 1 cup brown sugar
- Two chia eggs (2 tbsp. ground chia seeds + 4 tbsp. water)
- 1/4 cup all-purpose flour
- 1/4 cup coconut flour
- 1/2 cup cocoa powder
- 1/2 cup dark chocolate chips
- A pinch of grated nutmeg
- A bit of sea salt
- 2 tbsp. coconut milk

## Directions:

1. Start by preheating your Air Fryer to 340 degrees F. Now, spritz the sides and bottom of a baking pan with a nonstick cooking spray.

2. In a mixing bowl, beat the coconut oil and brown sugar until fluffy. Next, fold in the chia eggs and beat again until well combined.

3. After that, add in the remaining ingredients. Mix until everything is well incorporated.

4. Bake in the preheated Air Fryer for 20 minutes. Enjoy!

## Nutrition:

279 Calories

20.8g Fat

25.8g Carbs

2.9g Protein

2.5g Fiber

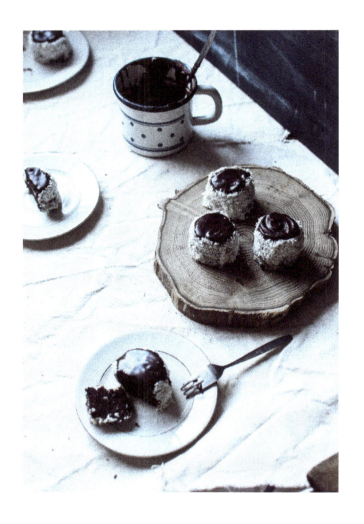

# 24.    Easy Apple Pie

Preparation Time: 5 minutes

Cooking Time: 35 minutes

Servings: 4

**Ingredients:**

- 12 ounces refrigerated two pie crusts

- 3 cups apples, peeled and thinly sliced

- 1/4 cup brown sugar

- tbsp. lemon juice

- 1 tsp. pure vanilla extract

- 1/2 tsp. cinnamon

- A pinch of ground cardamom

- A bit of kosher salt

**Directions:**

1. Place the first pie crust on a lightly greased pie plate.

2. In a mixing bowl, thoroughly combine the remaining ingredients to make the filling. Spoon

the filling into the pie crust that has been prepared.

3. Unroll the second pie crust and place it on top of the filling.

4. Bake the apple pie at 350 degrees F for 35 minutes or until the top is golden brown. Bon appétit!

## Nutrition:

450 Calories

21.8g Fat

61.6g Carbs

2.7g Protein

3.7g Fiber

# 25.    Classic Homemade Beignets

Preparation Time: 10 minutes

Cooking Time: 10 minutes

Servings: 4

**Ingredients:**

- 3/4 cup all-purpose flour

- tsp. baking powder

- 1/4 tsp. kosher salt

- 1/4 cup yogurt

- Two eggs, beaten

- 1/4 cup granulated sugar

- 2 tbsp. coconut oil, melted

**Directions:**

1. In a prepared mixing bowl, thoroughly combine all the ingredients.

2. Drop a spoonful of batter onto the greased Air Fryer pan. Cook in the preheated Air Fryer at 360

degrees F for 10 minutes, flipping them halfway through the cooking time.

3. Repeat with the remaining batter and then serve warm. Enjoy!

## Nutrition:

250 Calories

12.8g Fat

25.6g Carbs

7.7g Protein

# 26.    Classic Chocolate Cupcakes

Preparation Time: 5 minutes

Cooking Time: 15 minutes

Servings: 6

**Ingredients:**

- 3/4 cup all-purpose flour
- 1 tsp. baking powder
- 1/4 tsp. ground cinnamon
- 1/4 tsp. ground cardamom
- 3/4 cup granulated sugar
- 1/4 cups unsweetened cocoa powder
- A pinch of sea salt
- stick butter at room temperature
- 3/4 cup milk
- eggs, beaten

## Directions:

1. Preheat your Air Fryer set the temperature to 330 degrees F.

2. Mix all the ingredients in a bowl. Scrape the batter into silicone baking molds; place them in the Air Fryer basket.

3. Bake your cupcakes for 15 minutes or until a tester comes out dry and clean.

4. Allow the cupcakes to cool before unmolding and serving. Bon appétit!

## Nutrition:

337 Calories

18g Fat

40.6g Carbs

5.5g Protein

# 27. Southern-Style Peaches

Preparation Time: 5 minutes

Cooking Time: 15 minutes

Servings: 4

**Ingredients:**

- Three peaches halved
- 1 tbsp. fresh lime juice
- 1/2 tsp. ground cinnamon
- 1/2 tsp. grated nutmeg
- 1/2 cup brown sugar
- 4 tbsp. coconut oil

**Directions:**

1. Toss the peaches with the remaining ingredients.
2. Pour 1/4 cup of water into an Air Fryer safe dish. Place the peaches in the dish.
3. Bake the peaches at 340 degrees F for 15 minutes. Serve at room temperature. Bon appétit!

## **Nutrition:**

280 Calories

18.8g Fat

31.8g Carbs

1.4g Protein

# 28.    Favorite Fudge Cake

Preparation Time: 5 minutes

Cooking Time: 20 minutes

Servings: 5

## Ingredients:

- 1/2 cup butter, melted
- 1 cup turbinado sugar
- Three eggs
- tsp. vanilla extract
- 1/4 tsp. salt
- 1/4 tsp. ground cloves
- 1/2 tsp. ground cinnamon
- 1/2 cup all-purpose flour
- 1/4 cup almond flour
- 5 ounces chocolate chips

## Directions:

1. Start by preheating your Air Fryer to 340 degrees F. Now, spritz the sides and bottom of a baking pan with a nonstick cooking spray.

2. In a prepared mixing bowl, beat the butter and sugar until fluffy. Next, fold in the eggs and beat again until well combined.

3. After that, add in the remaining ingredients. Mix until everything is well combined.

4. Bake in the preheated Air Fryer for 20 minutes. Enjoy!

## Nutrition:

431 Calories

23.8g Fat

49.5g Carbs

6.6g Protein

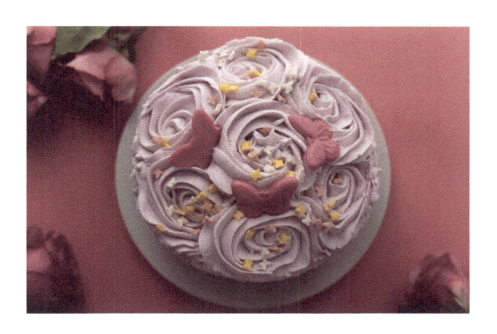

# 29.  Cinnamon Apple Wedges

Preparation Time: 3 minutes

Cooking Time: 17 minutes

Servings: 4

## Ingredients:

- Four apples, peeled, cored, and cut into wedges

- 2 tsp. coconut oil

- 3 tbsp. brown sugar

- 1 tsp. pure vanilla extract

- 1 tsp. ground cinnamon

- 1/4 cup water

## Directions:

1. Toss the apples with coconut oil, sugar, vanilla, and cinnamon.

2. Pour 1/4 cup of water into an Air Fryer safe dish. Place the apples in the dish.

3. Bake the apples at 340 degrees F for 17 minutes. Serve at room temperature. Bon appétit!

## Nutrition:

174 Calories

4.8g Fat

34.5g Carbs

0.6g Protein

# 30.  Old-Fashioned Pumpkin Cake

Preparation Time: 7 minutes

Cooking Time: 13 minutes

Servings: 4

## Ingredients:

- 1/2 cup pumpkin puree

- 1/2 cup peanut butter

- Four eggs, beaten

- 1 tsp. vanilla extract

- 1 tsp. pumpkin pie spice

- 1/2 tsp. baking powder

## Directions:

1. Mix all the ingredients to make the batter. Pour the batter into a lightly oiled baking pan.

2. Place the pan in the Air Fryer cooking basket.

3. Bake your cake at 350 degrees F for about 13 minutes or until it is golden brown around the edges. Bon appétit!

**Nutrition:**

269 Calories

15.8g Fat

20.5g Carbs

10.6g Protein

# 31.    Fluffy Scones with Cranberries

Preparation Time: 3 minutes

Cooking Time: 17 minutes

Servings: 4

**Ingredients:**

- 1 cup all-purpose flour

- 1 tsp. baking powder

- 1/4 cup caster sugar

- A pinch of sea salt

- 1/4 tsp. ground cinnamon

- 4 tbsp. butter

- egg, beaten

- 1/4 cup milk

- ounces dried cranberries

## Directions:

1. Preheat your Air Fryer set the temperature to 360 degrees F.

2. Mix all the ingredients until everything is well incorporated. Spoon the batter into baking cups; lower the cups into the Air Fryer basket.

3. Bake your scones for about 17 minutes or until a tester comes out dry and clean. Bon appétit!

## Nutrition:

326 Calories

14.8g Fat

42.5g Carbs

6g Protein

# 32.    Grilled Plantain Boats

Preparation Time: 5 minutes

Cooking Time: 7 minutes

Servings: 4

**Ingredients:**

- Four plantains, peeled

- 1/2 cup coconut, shredded

- 1 tbsp. coconut oil

- 4 tbsp. brown sugar

- 1/2 tsp. cinnamon powder

- 1/2 tsp. cardamom powder

- 4 tbsp. raisins

**Directions:**

1. In the peel, slice your plantains lengthwise; make sure not to cut all the way through the plantains.

2. Divide the remaining ingredients between the plantain pockets.

3. Place the plantain boats in the Air Fryer grill pan.

   Cook at 395 degrees F for 7 minutes.

4. Eat with a spoon and enjoy!

## Nutrition:

354 Calories

7.6g Fat

74.5g Carbs

2.8g Protein

# 33.   Almond Chocolate Cake

Preparation Time: 5 minutes

Cooking Time: 20 minutes

Servings: 6

## Ingredients:

- One stick butter, melted

- 1/2 cups brown sugar

- Two eggs, at room temperature

- 5 ounces chocolate chips

- 1/2 tsp. pure vanilla extract

- 1/2 tsp. pure almond extract

- 1/4 cup cocoa powder (Note 3)1/4 cup cocoa powder (Note 3)

- 1/4 cup all-purpose flour

- 1/2 cup almond flour

- 1/2 tsp. baking powder

- 2 ounces almonds, slivered

- 4 tbsp. coconut milk

## Directions:

1. Start by preheating your Air Fryer to 340 degrees F. Then, brush the sides and bottom of a baking pan with a nonstick cooking spray.

2. In a prepared mixing bowl, beat the butter and sugar until fluffy. Next, fold in the eggs and beat again until well combined.

3. After that, add in the remaining ingredients. Mix until everything is well combined.

4. Bake in the preheated Air Fryer for 20 minutes. Enjoy!

## Nutrition:

344 Calories

22.8g Fat

32.5g Carbs

6g Protein

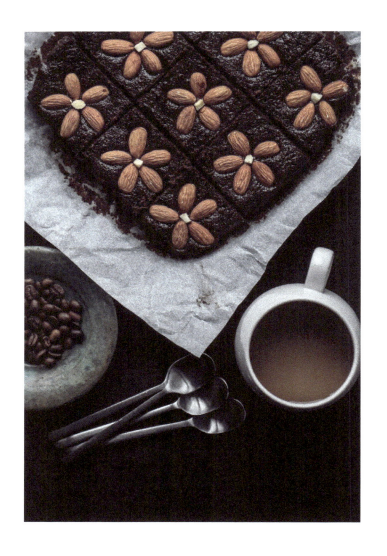

# 34.　Classic Fried Plums

Preparation Time: 3 minutes

Cooking Time: 17 minutes

Servings: 4

**Ingredients:**

- 1 pound plums, halved and pitted

- 2 tbsp. coconut oil

- 4 tbsp. brown sugar

- Four whole cloves

- One cinnamon stick

- Four whole stars anise

**Directions:**

1. Toss the plums with the remaining ingredients.

2. Pour 1/4 cup of water into an Air Fryer safe dish. Place the plums in the dish.

3. Bake the plums at 340 degrees F for 17 minutes. Serve at room temperature. Bon appétit!

**Nutrition:**

144 Calories

7.2g Fat

20.9g Carbs

0.7g Protein

# 35.    Classic Cinnamon Donuts

Preparation Time: 10 minutes

Cooking Time: 10 minutes

Servings: 4

**Ingredients:**

- 12 ounces large flaky biscuits

- 1/4 cup granulated sugar

- 1 tsp. ground cinnamon

- 1/4 tsp. grated nutmeg

- 2 tbsp. coconut oil

**Directions:**

1. Separate the dough into biscuits and place them in a lightly oiled Air Fryer cooking basket.

2. Mix the sugar, cinnamon, nutmeg, and coconut oil until well combined.

3. Drizzle your donuts with the cinnamon mixture.

4. Bake your donuts in the preheated Air Fryer at 340 degrees F for approximately 10 minutes or

until golden. Repeat with the remaining donuts.

Bon appétit!

## Nutrition:

374 Calories

16.2g Fat

52.1g Carbs

5.5g Protein

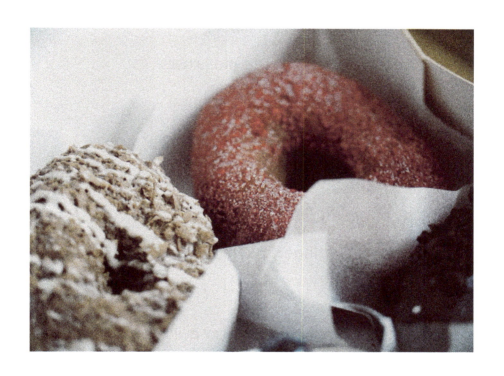

# 36.  Classic Autumn Pie

Preparation Time: 5 minutes

Cooking Time: 35 minutes

Servings: 4

## Ingredients:

- 12 ounces refrigerated pie crusts

- 1/2 cup pumpkin puree, canned

- 1-ounce walnuts, coarsely chopped

- 1/2 cup granulated sugar

- tsp. pumpkin pie spice mix

- 1 tsp. fresh ginger, peeled and grated

## Directions:

1. Place the first pie crust on a lightly greased pie plate.

2. In a mixing bowl, thoroughly combine the remaining ingredients to make the filling. Spoon the filling into the pie crust that has been prepared.

3. Unroll the second pie crust and place it on top of the filling.

4. Bake the pie set the temperature at 350 degrees F for 35 minutes or until the top is golden brown. Bon appétit!

## Nutrition:

534 Calories

26.4g Fat

72.3g Carbs

3.9g Protein

# 37.  Traditional Thai Goreng Pisang

Preparation Time: 7 minutes

Cooking Time: 13 minutes

Servings: 4

**Ingredients:**

- 8 tbsp. rice flour

- 8 tbsp. all-purpose flour

- 1/4 tsp. ground cinnamon

- A pinch of sea salt

- A bit of grated nutmeg

- 8 tbsp. coconut flakes

- 3 tsp. coconut oil

- Four eggs whisked

- Four bananas, peeled and sliced

## Directions:

1. Preheat your Air Fryer set the temperature to 390 degrees F.

2. In a mixing dish, thoroughly combine the flour, cinnamon, salt, nutmeg, and coconut flakes.

3. Now, add in the coconut oil and eggs. Roll each slice of banana over the egg/flour mixture.

4. Bake your bananas in the preheated Air Fryer for approximately 13 minutes, turning them over halfway through the cooking time. Bon appétit!

## Nutrition:

384 Calories

12.2g Fat

60.8g Carbs

18.7g Protein

# 38.    Easy French Dessert

Preparation Time: 10 minutes

Cooking Time: 10 minutes

Servings: 4

## Ingredients:

- Four eggs

- 3 tbsp. coconut oil, melted

- 1/2 cup milk

- 1/2 tsp. vanilla extract

- 1/4 tsp. ground cinnamon

- 1/8 tsp. ground nutmeg

- Eight thick slices of baguette

## Directions:

1. In a mixing bowl, thoroughly combine the eggs, coconut oil, milk, vanilla, cinnamon, and nutmeg.

2. Then, dip each piece of bread into the egg mixture; place the bread slices in a lightly greased baking pan.

3. Air Fryer the bread slices at 330 degrees F for about 4 minutes; turn them over and cook for 3 to 4 minutes. Enjoy!

**Nutrition:**

310 Calories

20.4g Fat

22.3g Carbs

9g Protein

# 39.  American-Style Crullers

Preparation Time: 10 minutes

Cooking Time: 10 minutes

Servings: 4

**Ingredients:**

- 3/4 cup all-purpose flour

- 1/4 cup butter

- 1/4 cup water

- 1/2 cup full-fat milk

- 1/4 tsp. kosher salt

- A pinch of grated nutmeg

- Three eggs, beaten

**Directions:**

1. In a prepared mixing bowl, thoroughly combine all ingredients. Place the batter in a piping bag fitted with a large open star tip.

2. Pipe your crullers into circles and lower them onto the greased Air Fryer pan.

3. Cook your crullers in the preheated Air Fryer at 360 degrees F for 10 minutes, flipping them halfway through the cooking time.

4. Repeat with the remaining batter then serve immediately. Enjoy!

**Nutrition:**

250 Calories

15.4g Fat

19.3g Carbs

7.9g Protein

## Conclusion:

Now that Air fryer ovens are no less than a kitchen miracle, but now it is your job to take care of your family and friends from further harm. What is an air fryer, and how can we use it? Air fryers are what you need to cook your food using little or no oil. Giving them healthier foods with the aromas of old meals is your mission. From now on, use the Air Fryer instead of traditional frying. Give yourself the best shape and health since you have the expertise. In this cookbook, the author has managed to share as many different recipes as to provide an extensive insight into the preparation of other delicious tasting meals. Try these out as a start. Maybe you will find the best recipe for the most healthy food you ever tasted. You know that frying is not good for your health, but you also love fried stuff. So, Air fryers are the best option for you. The biggest advantage of air fryers is that they use little to no oil. Any oil you want to use can be from a healthier oil option like extra virgin olive oil. Now you have enough information about air fryers and their benefits in cooking. You know that they are used all over the world and are popular among food lovers and chefs.

So, you can use the information and get a great deal on air fryers. You will be able to make fried foods

that are crispy and tasty without worrying about extra calories or harmful oils. Pick the best fryer for you and enjoy the new era of healthy fried food.

Both pans and pots are kitchen essentials. Each of these products has its purpose. As you know, pots are for cooking liquid food like soup and vegetables while skillets are for cooking solid food like meat. But the air fryer is like a pot that cooks food at the same time.

People like fried food. This is why lots of foods are fried at restaurants like fried chicken, fish, and burgers. But you have tried all these kinds of foods, but still, you crave unhealthy and fatty food. Now you need fried healthy food; that is why you have to use the air fryer. It is kitchen enlightenment. You can cook both the meat and vegetables in one fryer. In fact, it preserves the healthy fats present in the foods while suppressing the unhealthy fats. Your food will be hard on the outside but soft on the inside. You will be able to eat fried stuff without feeling guilty. You can start your morning with a healthy breakfast of eggs cooked in your air fryer. Make these foods without having to worry about your health. Try the new recipes shared in this cookbook.

Its air fryer recommendations will help you get the best products that will last for long. Your food will be fried just the way you like it. The air fryer will preserve the healthy fats present in the food while suppressing the unhealthy fats. You do not have to worry about the calories present in the food because of the low use of oil. You will get the best results and will enjoy your fried food all the time.